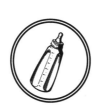

Congratulations Allen & Debi!   June 17, 1994

   Amy & I are so excited for you. Having seen some approximation of what you will be going through next year ourselves. We know you will have a great time. There are lows and there are highs, but they both make the journey all the more worthwhile.

   Please make sure to let us know how things are going & don't hesitate to call for advice or a kind word.

                         Love
                         Mark & Amy

PS: Take this gift with the proverbial "grain of salt". It ain't all that bad!

Allen & Debi—
Your news was the best this month! The world definitely could use a person with both your qualities. Debi, although the fear of the "unknown" can be a bit overwhelming, I am a bit sad

Before &After

Your New Baby

by
Victoria Brown and Allan Chochinov

that I will never walk that path
or the first time again. There is
something really neat about that
nervousness and excitement. I love
being a Mom... although I drink a lot
more wine these days! Congrats! Amy

ST. MARTIN'S PRESS • NEW YORK

BEFORE & AFTER™—YOUR NEW BABY

ISBN: 0-312-95339-9

Before & After is the exclusive trademark of
Victoria Brown and Allan Chochinov

Book and cover design: Victoria Brown and Allan Chochinov
Authors' photo: John Carroll

Printed in the United States of America

St. Martin's Paperbacks edition / May 1994

10 9 8 7 6 5 4 3 2 1

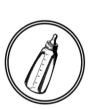

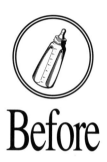

Before

"I feel so young to be having a baby."

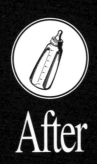

After

"Wow, am I too old for this."

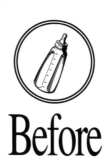

Before

cut the cake

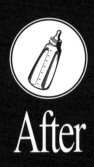

After

cut the cord

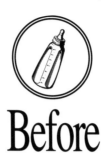

Before

Democrat or Republican?

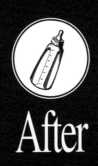

After

inny or outy?

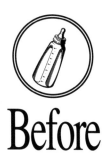

Before

"The Joy of Sex"

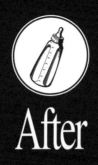

After

"What to Expect When You're Expecting"

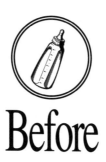

Before

"Yeah, they said their baby was cute,
but *all* babies are cute."

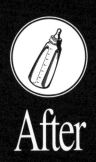

After

"Ours *is the most beautiful.*"

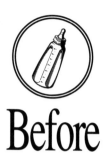

Before

Wall Street

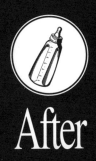

After

Sesame Street

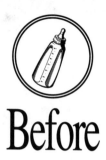

Before

searching for a dressing room

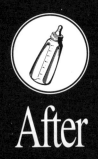

After

searching for a changing room

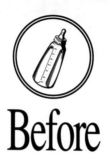

Before

goo-goo eyes

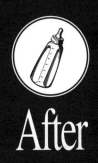

After

ga-ga goo-goo

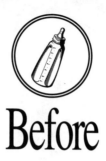

Before

"I want her to learn the value of a dollar."

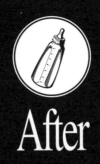

After

*"Yes, I'll take that doll, these books, and that set of blocks.
And don't forget the hobby horse.
Oh, and that model train too, please."*

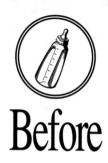

Before

Coming Soon

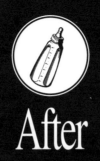

After

Now Showing

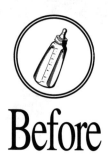

Before

bungee jumper

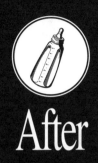

After

Jolly Jumper

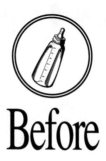

Before

"You're always calling your mother."

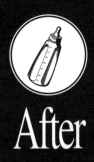

After

"Maybe you could call your mother for tonight?"

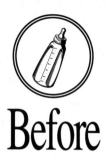

Before

high heels

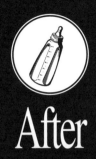

After

high chair

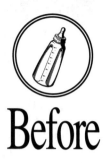

Before

"Douglas and I are very fussy about the objects we choose
for our apartment. Nothing gaudy, very little color."

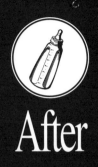

After

"I come home, and it looks like a Toys 'R' Us delivery truck crashed into our living room."

Before

O-B-G-Y-N

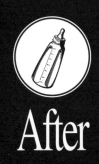

After

M-O-U-S-E

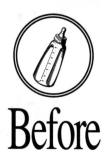

Before

Sugar and spice and everything nice

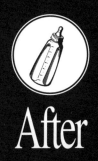

After

"Sugar makes him crazy, and spices give him gas."

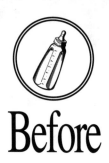

Before

teddy

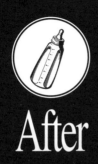

After

Teddy

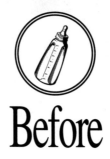

Before

"And she brought that little terror to the office.
I couldn't get a minute's work done."

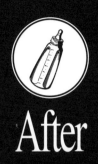

After

"You guys don't mind if I set up her Perky PlayPen next to the coffee counter, do you?"

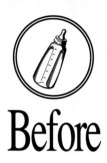

Before

diamond ring

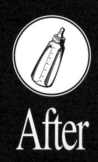

After

teething ring

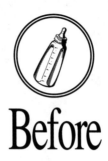

Before

"No, really, honey—you go out with the boys tonight.
I'll be fine here on my own."

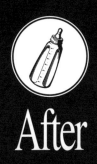

After

*"How could you have gone out tonight
and left me all alone with that little monster?!"*

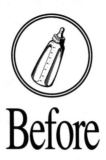

Before

a splash of perfume on your wrist

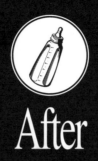

After

a splash of milk on your wrist

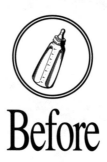

Before

rob the cradle

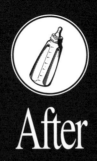

After

rock the cradle

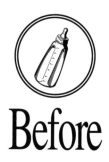

Before

"Lars gazed greedily at Felicia
as the fire in his loins began to gnaw at him."

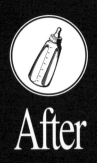

After

"Once upon a time, there were three little bears."

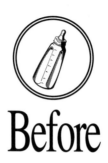

Before

garters

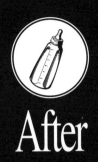

After

Gerbers

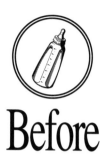

Before

"We will share parenting equally."

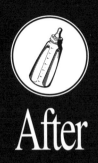

After

"You're *his mother. DO something!*"

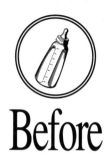

Before

Mr. Spock

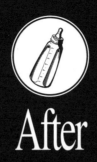

After

Dr. Spock

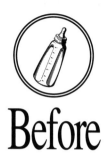

Before

"I don't understand why parents worry so
much about leaving their baby with a sitter.
I mean, what could possibly happen?"

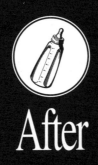

After

"*And here are the numbers to the fire department, the police station, the poison control unit, and the emergency room. The SWAT Command Center and the radon hot line are programmed into the speed dial.*"

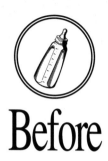

Before

dinner parties

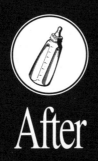

After

birthday parties

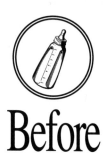

Before

Stain-Blaster Ultra Bleach
with Dirt-Crusher Killer Enzymes

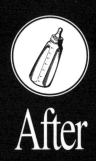

After

Ivory Snow

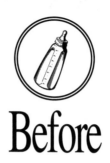

Before

single

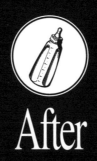

After

"Twins!"

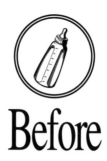

Before

"Mike never goes anywhere without his cellular phone."

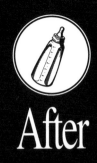

After

"Mike never goes anywhere without the camcorder."

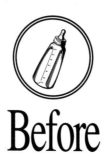

Before

swollen ankles

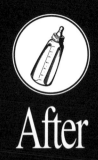

After

swollen credit

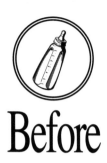

Before

daiquiris in a blender

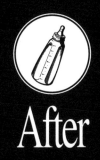

After

peas in a blender

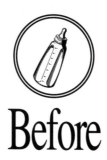

Before

"How could you think of
bringing a child into this world?"

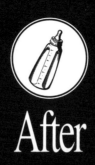

After

*"How could you think of
bringing a child into this movie theatre?"*

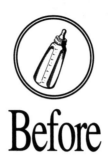

Before

night life

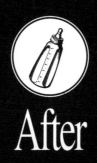

After

night light

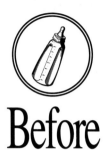

Before

"Don't try to change me."

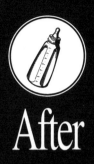

After

"Honey, it's your turn to change her."

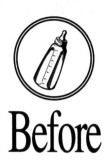

Before

push-up bra

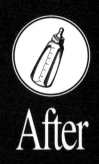

After

feeding bra

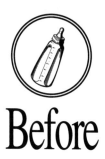

Before

be fruitful and multiply

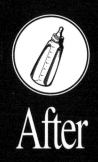

After

be fruitful and multiply your expenses by ten

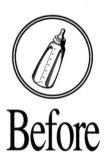

Before

the right firm

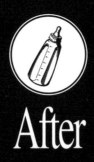

After

the right playgroup

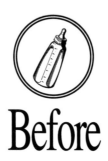

Before

"And it's going to be *totally* drug-free.
Period."

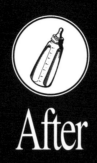

After

"GIVE ME MY EPIDURAL!
NOW!"

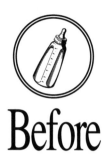

Before

"Baby, baby, oh baby."

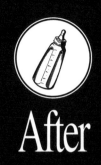

After

baby

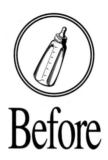

Before

bananas flambé

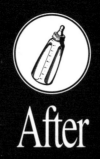

After

flying bananas

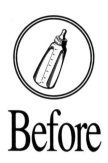

Before

"He's going to have *your* eyes and hair,
and *my* easy temperament."

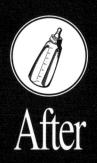

After

"Are you sure they didn't mix up the cribs?"

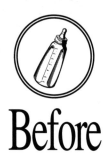

Before

last call

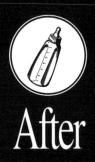

After

first feeding

With special thanks to our parents, Andrea & David and Ethel & Earl, without whom, of course, this book never would have been possible.